Get Off the Cow Now!

Written by Michael Foley

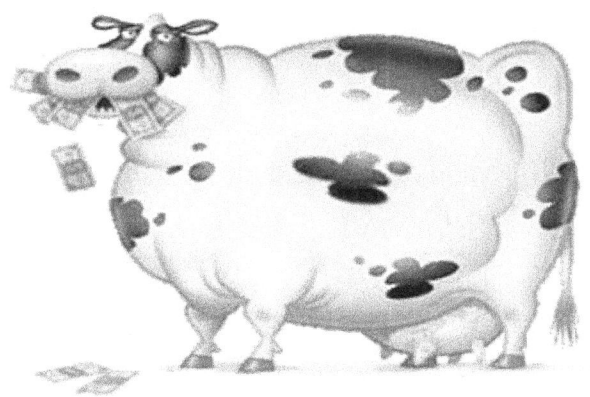

My Simple Cure for Cancer

It's simple and <u>easy</u>!

You will benefit from this book whether you have cancer or not, it just makes sense for everyone to start eating better.

If you have been told you don't have cancer, it's probably not showing up yet because it's too small. I strongly recommend you start eating right today before you <u>have</u> to!

A traditional medical screening can only "detect" cancer when it is roughly the size of a pea – a billion cancer cells – which they can see, scan, measure, and poke.

After Cancer found me in 2012, I started an alternative plan to heal my cancer naturally without surgery, radiation, or chemotherapy. I have conducted hundreds of hours of research and experimentation to come up with a compatible treatment plan that heals/prevents cancer naturally and effectively without the use of supplements or expensive fads.

You can achieve optimal health through a plant based eating arrangement and this book will show you how without a huge amount of aggravation.

This is not a diet . . .
"it's a new eating arrangement!"

Every bite you take is either
fighting disease
or feeding it.

Introduction

I'm Not a Writer . . . Not a Victim . . . I'm a cancer survivor/Flexitarian.

Cancer does not have to be a death sentence. Eating red meat and using dairy products are the **death** sentence, in my opinion.

Here are the problems with today's commercial cows, starting with the milk/dairy products. Fifty years ago an average cow produced **2,000 pounds/** 200 gallons of milk per year. Today the top producers produce **50,000 pounds/**5,000 gallons! This is accomplished with drugs, antibiotics, hormones, forced feeding plans and specialized breeding. A gallon of milk weighs about 10 pounds. When you drink a glass of milk it's like putting a pound of liquid in your body and some of it sticks.

To begin this wonderful journey, I'm suggesting you quit dairy products for seven days. Dairy products are those foods made from milk including: Cream, Cheese, Milk, Yogurt, Ice Cream, Butter, Sour Cream, Buttermilk, Creme Fraiche, Clotted Cream, Condensed Milk, Evaporated Milk, Chocolate Milk, Skim Milk, No Fat Milk, all milk. I have had quite a few people ask if no fat milk is included because it's almost water. The answer is milk is milk unless it's an almond or soymilk. When you quit dairy products for seven days you will expel about a gallon of mucus from your kidneys, spleen, pancreas, and other internal organs. This is what I mean by some of it sticks.

Your one-week experience will be as if an internal fog has been dispersed from inside of you. Most people who successfully wean themselves from all milk and dairy products immediately observe dramatic physical and emotional changes. Better sleep, more energy, fewer mood swings, more sexual energy. Source: Notmilk.com

If you stop just the milk, it's a great start and its just milk. You might try replacing it with almond, coconut, rice or soymilk. It's actually delicious. After one week of not consuming dairy products and reading the information below, you won't want it anymore. Ultimately you will stop all dairy products . . . you'll feel better and lose weight. The Dairy products are the beginning, next is the sugar.

I suggest you start a journal right now and write down what you have ingested for the last couple of days and continue documenting this for as long as you can. This will help immensely later in this book.

I am not a medical professional and all information given in this book is for informational purposes only and should be used at your own risk.

TABLE OF CONTENTS

Chapter 1
Getting to Know Me

I went to a highly referred wellness Doctor and had a full blood test for the first time in 10 years. One week later, we sat down and discussed the results. He said "you're in very good condition, however, your PSA (prostate specific antigen) is measured at 125 when it should be less than 5. Immediately we set an appointment with a proctologist for a biopsy of the prostate.

I was diagnosed with prostrate cancer on October 19, 2012 with a Gleason score of 7 (3+4). A Gleason score of 2 to 4 means the cells still look very much like normal cells and pose little danger of spreading quickly. A score of 5 to 7 indicates intermediate risk. A score of 8 to 10 indicates that the cells have very few features of a normal cell and are likely to be aggressive.

After being advised over the phone of my diagnosis, we (The Proctologist and I) scheduled an appointment to discuss the options. He advised me to bring a loved one. When the three of us sat down, he explained approximately 5 options, but to narrow it down I had to have another test. I asked why I didn't have the other test before this meeting. I guess it was an oversight because he was embarrassed to admit it. I said, "let me get this straight. I go get the test and come back, bring my loved one (we are both on a very tight schedule) and pay you another $200?" He agreed that's what I needed to do. As we walked out I was thinking, "this is the last time I walk through this door ever again".

Now, I'm thinking "options". So, I went straight to the Wellness Doctor and he recommended a Holistic method. I for one like to push the envelope in my life, so I tried his way of curing myself of this prostate cancer stuff. This did not include Chemo, radiation or a prostatectomy, pronounced (pros·ta·tec·to·my) which is the surgical removal of the prostate gland.

I was told I had to have this prostatectomy as the cure if the PET Scan came back negative; meaning has not already spread throughout my body.

By the way . . . the chance of Erectile Dysfunction from the removal of the prostrate is very, very, very high. Statistics show a 50/50 chance. We are **all** too young for that.

Source:
http://www.sharecare.com/health/erectile-dysfunction/how-common-ed-prostate-cancer

By choosing the Holistic Method, the result now two years later . . . (Drum Roll Please) . . . I am still alive . . . healthy (Bada Bing) and happier (Bada Boom) than I was the day I was diagnosed with this deadly disease.

I believe life is like a game of golf. You have to play the ball where it lies.

This book is just my opinion; the results have spoken for themselves. I am not a Doctor, (though I have been called one) so don't forget it is just my opinion. All I know is it's working for me and working for many other people. Check it out for yourself. Research how many people slowed down or stopped cancer through Holistic/ Naturopathic methods as opposed to Chemo, Radi or Snip n' Snip . . . and I saved money!

The reason why I wrote this book is to heighten your awareness and teach you the types of discipline it takes to get through this gracefully.

Discipline is the key factor regarding this method

and it's a real pain in the south side of a northbound mule, to say the least.

"it's a new eating arrangement"

Chemo wasn't an option for me. However, the Average Cost of Cancer Chemotherapy is as follows:

The cost of eight weeks of chemotherapy can range from $100 to $30,000. Treatment with inexpensive drugs like 5-FU or leucovorin costs around $300 dollars for eight weeks. However, to improve therapeutic effect, these drugs are often used in combination with newer drugs, which are typically more expensive. According to Johns Hopkins Health Alerts, addition of Avastin® or Erbitux® to 5-FU or leucovorin can push up the cost of the dosing regimen to as much as $30,000.

Source: http://www.livestrong.com/article/153376-the-average-cost-for-cancer-chemotherapy-treatment/

Vast majority of Oncologists would not use Chemotherapy if they got cancer themselves. Read more on this unbelievable subject:

http://www.cancerresearchinformation.com/vast-majority-of-oncologists-would-not-use-chemotherapy-if-they-got-cancer/#ixzz3KhdsOma0

With the holistic method, now my method, you will "Save Money".

How the heck did you do that you ask? Well, I'll tell Ya Pilgrim!

I am going to request that you begin with a 50% vegetarian/Flexitarian method. Next time you are at the grocery store look at the price of a good steak compared to the price of a head of lettuce. You do the math.

Things that many people fail to think through are the facts that some of the foods that you eat may actually be causing the problems that you are having. Hence, Get Off The Cow Now!

It goes without saying that a diet loaded with fatty fried foods or those rich in additives and preservatives aren't good for you. Not only can they cause you to feel run down, but they can also ensure that your body won't work properly. This can contribute to the development of a common cold or even make your joints hurt. There may also be foods that you eat that you are actually allergic

13

to without even realizing it. These may cause the allergic reaction that you are familiar with and therefore, you want to do your part to really analyze your diet. This is why the food journal is so important. Foods that are harmful include wheat, gluten, sugar, and dairy products.

In the past before my new arrangement with food intake, if my joints hurt I'd take a pill, run down, take a pill, allergic reaction . . . take a pill. Now because of my "new eating arrangement", my joints don't hurt, I'm not run down, my allergies are non-existent, my blood pressure is stable and I don't take blood pressure pills anymore. Thanks to my Naturopathic Doctor

Keep in mind . . .

Small Changes That Make Big Differences

Chapter 2 –

My Naturopathic Doctor

When my Wellness/Naturopathic Doctor suggested I go 90% vegetarian I said "Whaaaaaaaa . . ." like the guy on Matt Damon's Water Commercial

http://www.metatube.com/en/videos/171522/Interview-Matt-Damon-Goes-On-Strike-Water/

I then replied, "sure I can do 90%" (I was expecting 100%). His advice to me was "no more Meat, Dairy, Wheat, Sugar, Beer and Whiskey". I responded, "get the heck outta' town, Mista". He laughed and said, "you don't have to unless you want to get rid of your cancer and stop your joint pain". Remembering to "keep my humor", I thought, I'll show that "bag of nonsense".

I broke the news to him . . . "I'm Irish". I've enjoyed beer and whiskey all of my adult life, so it's a **habit**. He suggested I replace Whiskey with Tequila. "You can drink as much Tequila as you want. It's a plant base pure liquor that won't hurt you and stop the beer".

Basically, one thing you want to look for on the

bottle of Tequila is that it is "100% de Agave". What this means is that all the alcohol contained within the bottle is a direct result of the fermentation of the agave and only the agave; no sugar or other additives have been included to supplement the creation of the alcohol. In the end, this results in better tasting tequila and hopefully no hangovers.

So being quite the negotiator that I thought I was... I said, "Ok, Ok, Ok... I can change to Tequila and cut my beer in half" His response was outstandingly priceless . . . he said . . . "OK" with a friendly smile.

I responded, "a few beers a week is not going to make that big of difference". "No Problem" was his response. At that moment I felt like "he won". However, in actuality come to find out, I won, because I listened to him and today I am a different person and still creating the ultimate health, spiritual wealth & happiness.

I started to leave his office with my head hung low and my tail betweenst my legs. I said to one of the girls "No Milk, No Cookies, No Beer, No Whiskey. No Bueno". She said, "try Almond Milk, it's not bad and there is a book out there, a New York Times best-selling author and wellness activist, who convinced me to give up milk". So, I said "OK" thinking to myself whatever. I'm gonna' go get me a shot of that there "Ta-kill-ya" and a beer!

Ecstatic I was not to say the least with this new arrangement. Remembering the humor part, I thought to myself . . . I'll show that "bag of nonsense", I'll buy (and read) that book and quit consuming all the good stuff I used to eat.

I bought the eBook that night.

What I learned transformed my life forever – now it can transform yours. Of course, with a twist of the Foley.

I highly recommend Wellness Doctors. After you read this book . . . you might . . . no . . . you will . . . become very upset during the next 21 to 1,000 days still wanting all that you have had in the past. Myself, I became a real butthead to the point I was a miserable recluse. Now that I've made it through the tough part, I decided to write this book to get **"YOU"** prepared for the actual craziness you might go through without the knowledge from this book.

My problem was being able to read what my body was telling me without misinterpreting it, which I used to do a lot. You have to remind yourself daily that you will survive by changing almost all the things you have indulged and enjoyed your whole entire life and come out of it with a great big smile.

Before the new eating arrangement, I was working with a young lady who is a vegan. When all of us went to lunch, she would bring her own "stuff in a tub" is what I called it. I kinda' gave her a few jabs about it in jest. Since then, I have communicated to her that I am vegetable eating fool and feel soooo much better and I'm a Wellness Warrior/ Flexitarian. Flexitarian is a vegetarian that eats meat once in awhile.

By the way . . . I'm kidding about the "bag of nonsense" he is a great man that I respect dearly

What is Naturopathic Medicine?

Naturopathic medicine is based on the belief that the human body has an innate healing ability. Naturopathic doctors teach their patients to use diet, exercise, lifestyle changes and natural therapies to enhance their bodies and the ability to ward off and combat disease, but to also restore health.

If you are serious about changing your life . . .

18

The **Time is NOW!**

Also, don't stop at this book. Keep asking questions on the Internet regarding every bite you take, it'll surprise you!

Chapter 3 –

Plant-Power Arrangement

A Plant-power diet can reap huge health benefits.

Juicy tomatoes, sweet peaches, sizzling peppers . . . summer produce is a great way for you to get all the benefits that a plant based diet offers. And here's the latest proof that it can help your heart grow younger.

In a study from the Cleveland clinic (where Dr. Mike Roizen is chief wellness officer; he's also co-author of the study), 198 Women and men with heart disease stayed on a produce-packed, plant-based diet for 3 1/2 years. They gave up processed foods, along with added sugars and salt, meat, poultry even fish, vegetable oils and caffeine. On their plates: loads of artery-pampering leafy greens, plus plenty of hearty whole grains, satisfying beans and heaping helpings of fruit and veggies.

It was a huge diet overhaul for the study volunteers, and an impressive 89% stuck with it. A whopping 94% of those who stayed on the plant diet saw symptoms as chest pain reduced. Just one person from that group suffered a health event related to artery disease (a stroke). In contrast, during the course of the study, 62% of those who didn't stick with the diet-experienced event, including stroke, artery-clearing or bypass surgery and heart related death.

To start reaping the delicious benefits of plant-based eating, start with the small yet powerful changes:

Quit eating fast foods, personally I still have to have a burger once in awhile, like once a month. Banish foods packed with saturated fat, trans fat, added sodium, sweeteners, syrups and all dairy products.

Eat leafy greens every day.

Salad, a side dish of sautéed kale, collards, spinach or chard, a green smoothie . . . find new ways to fit a variety of greens. Start the day with fruit.

Source: Mehmet Oz, MD and Mike Roizen

Chapter 4 –

The Knockout Punch

What I mean by The Knockout Punch is some people, including myself, have to be punched in the nose and knocked to ground before they will listen. In the next chapters I will help you up, dust you off and clean yourself up, in a good way.

If you want to try my method, please check with your new Wellness Doctor (if you don't have a Wellness Doctor, it's time to find your own local personal hero) to see if there will be any adverse consequences/reactions before you try this. I did and I'm glad I did.

I think about what my Grandparent's ate and how they lived into there 90's. Here's what I've learned and want to share:

1. **We all have Cancer**.

2. We can cure cancer this year! Only if you want to.

3. A good start is to stop raising God's children/animals to slaughter and eat. It's called supply and demand.

4. Stop consuming all dairy products. Try almond milk, I did. That's now what I drink when I want a glass of milk. No CHEESE, sorry. For me in the past, it was a big glass of two percent milk and a bunch of cookies. Now it's Broccoli dipped in Honey Mustard, and big ol' glass of water!

5. Stop consuming all wheat products. There's a lot of wheat in bread & beer . . . sorry.

6. Stop consuming sugar, again . . . sorry.

7. Start at 50% then work toward 90% plant-based eating arrangement and drink more water with a high pH value.

8. Humor . . . lot's and lot's of Humor. Do you know the difference between humor and odor? Humor is just a shift of wit, and odor is just a

whiff of . .

9. If you smoke cigarettes . . . quit!!! I quit. Please
don't try to quit until you really want to.
Otherwise, you're wasting your time and energy
and it's depressing. Depression is very bad for you.
Positive thinking is very good for you. Just know
you will positively quit someday soon.

This is how to enjoy your food without going
insane, starting with breakfast.

Breakfast:

I used to be an egg, bacon, waffle or cereal and
toast with lots n' lots of butter and blueberry jam,
every day kinda' of person. Now breakfast consists
of (IMAGINE THIS) a "Chocolate Milkshake" made
with CHOCOLATE almond milk, strawberries,
bananas and beets. You name it, as long as it tastes
good and is plant-based stuff only 90% of the
time!

Remember the "tastes good" part is very important
because at one point I said to my Doctor "I tried
Tofu and I had that gagging effect as I ate it" he
said, "then don't eat it. There are so many things
out there that are meat substitutes you might find
you like". So, the moral of this story is eat what's

good and don't eat what's bad. Simple, huh . . .

I searched the Internet for "meat substitutes for vegetarians" and a plethora of food items came up that are very good and to my surprise gives you that full feeling. Remember, you might have been brought up to think a full stomach is a happy stomach . . . wrong.

"The sleep of the working man is pleasant, whether he eats little or much; but the full stomach of the rich man does not allow him to sleep". – Ecclesiastes 5:12

I call this reprogramming your conditioned habits or de-brainwashing!

Then there is the time for cheating . . . yup . . . I CHEAT. It could be eggs-bacon-waffles, your call. Most importantly, enjoy that breakfast. **NO** guilt feelings. Enjoy it to the hilt because you're not going to get one for another 5 or 10 meals.

It's ok to cheat, but get back on that ol' wagon as soon as possible.

One thing to remember is if you cheat, you're feeding the cancer whom I call Jok. And by golly, I have a picture of Jok to share. Do you want to feed this guy? Jok will die if you don't feed him all the above items.

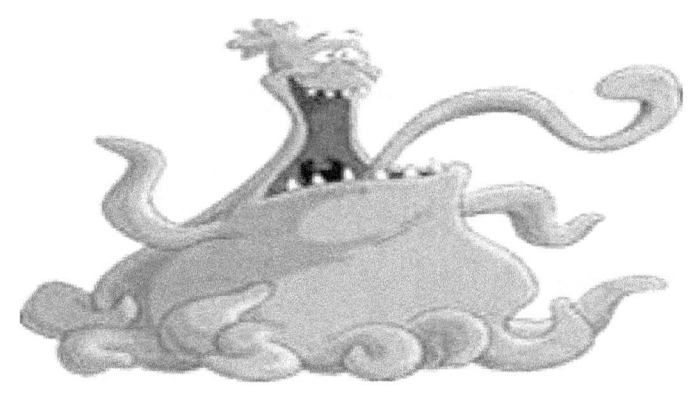

Jok (pronounced with a French accent)

My experience is when I cheat with let's say a Ding Dong. Before I consider driving to the store I say to myself "cheat with one Ding Dong . . . it's easier to cheat a second time". Then I'm hooked again on the 3rd and I have to start the process all over again. Please remember it's like playing Ping-Pong with cancer. As you know, you've never won all the Ping-Pong games you've played.

Sometimes I have to play Ping-Pong and get that Ding Dong, eat it and feel good about it.

Lunch:

I used to eat Roach Coach burritos or a drive-thru burger and fries. I did a job for a lady that told me at the very least eat at Subway. I replied, "I didn't have that kind of time". Now if I have to have a sandwich . . . it's a Subway sandwich. If I buy a loaf of bread . . . I'll eat it. The trick is to buy the loaf, take two slices for yourself and give the rest away.

No more fast food . . . sorry. Make a salad for work. Can you remember sitting at your desk an hour after lunch and falling asleep? This doesn't happen when you eat a plant food. When you dine out, just have the salad for lunch . . . no more burgers.

I made a decision to have anything I wanted every 10th meal. It works out very well in the long run because you get to flourish in the food you have waited nine meals for. Think of it as planning a mini vacation. In nine meals, I know I can have anything I want and savor that special moment.

Also . . . stay away from High Energy Drinks. They are loaded with lots and lots of sugar. A single Red Bull can increase your risk of a heart attack or stroke, whether you're young or old. It is loaded with caffeine and makes the blood sticky, which can be a pre-cursor to stroke and other cardiovascular problems. In just one hour after consuming a can of Red Bull, your blood can become as abnormal as someone with cardiovascular disease. Source: http://www.healthyfoodhouse.com/avoid-this-beverage-to-reduce-your-risk-of-having-a-stroke-and-heart-attack/

Dinner:

I was a steak, potatoes and a small salad, kinda' guy. Now, I fix a large salad with my favorite dressing on the side. Take a seat, start a movie and the next thing I know, the salad was delicious and I'm not full (your brain will grow accustom to the "not full" feeling). However, I'm not hungry either. So I always attempt to enjoy the movie and realize my brain and my stomach are satisfied. There is only one thing that I ask. The next time you have meat, just take a moment to appreciate that an animal gave its life for your meal. Now it's time for desert . . . Yay! Uh-Oh, what ever it was . . . change it. You might consider a fruit substitute. Only if you want to!

I have compiled a menu at the end of this book for

you to print and refer to which takes you from 50 to 80% Flexitarian.

There are so many sugar free cookies and things that will satisfy your craving. Personally, if I'm craving a candy bar or cookies I grab a glass of Chocolate Almond Milk or just go brush my teeth. Brushing your teeth, believe it or not, will suppress the craving for something sweet and cigarettes as well, if you are trying to quit.

Warning . . . you will get very tired, very quickly of salads. Spice them up by cooking one, two or three of the items in the salad. Such as the mushrooms, garlic and onions. Then, the salad is delicious and it becomes fun. It tricks your mind into thinking you had meat because you've cooked something.

Another alternative is to add lots of stuff . . . Avocados, Tomatoes, Raisins, Bananas, Cucumbers, etc. Don't worry about the sugar in the dressing, just put it on the side then dip. You automatically use less dressing when you dip. I have acquired a taste for honey mustard. Here is a simple recipe for it: http://www.wikihow.com/Make-Honey-Mustard

There comes a time when you _have_ to add meat to the salad . . . uh oh. No problem. Add some grilled chicken, shrimp or fish and enjoy the heck out of it. You might add a big ol' glass of wine or water remembering there is more sugar in wine then water. Oh wait; there isn't **any** sugar in water. But we know wine is better and that's OK!

There are many websites at your fingertips to join their daily e-mail lists regarding the right recipes. There are a lot of free ones to choose from.

It's not a diet . . . it's a new eating arrangement!

If you have meat, have 20% meat and 80% Veggies!

In the DVD "Forks over Knifes", the two doctors found a family of 8 in Asia would split a normal size steak, the same size I would normally consume by myself. They didn't have cancer years ago until the fast food restaurants came into play.

After one month of these new habits . . . okay maybe two months, I started feeling better with **"no"** more days of pain. To be relieved of all the joint pain was a miracle. The weight loss was a pleasant surprise.

The good news is these changes are free. You don't have to go out and buy anything. You may want to upgrade the cutting board and a few knifes.

Preparing your new foods is truly a new form of relaxation and a great feeling of meditation . . . only if you let it.

There **aren't** any miracle pills . . . just new habits.

Oh, by the way, here's another sweet little disturbing fact you probably didn't know about hamburgers and conventional beef: Chicken litter containing arsenic is fed to cows in factory beef operations. So the arsenic that's pooped out by the chickens gets consumed and concentrated in the tissues of cows, which is then ground into hamburger to be consumed by the clueless masses who don't even know they're eating second-hand chicken sh*t.

Source: http://www.healthy-holistic-living.com/fda-finally-admits-chicken-meat-contains-cancer-causing-arsenic.html?t=AHS

Stop! Take the time to smell your "new life". It is so refreshing to enjoy the moment. I can't tell you enough how important *Deep Breathing Exercise* is:
https://www.youtube.com/watch?v=g3k_-mciE6o

I'll keep reminding you of this newly formed habit you're going to acquire.

I used to be in a race with myself to see how much I could get accomplished in a day and wound up with high blood pressure (**hypertension**) and **cancer**. It's been almost 2 years since I began this new way of living and my PSA is down from 125 to 18 and my blood pressure is stabilized at a reasonable rate and I don't have to take pills any more. Regarding the blood pressure, we all have built in monitors if you listen to them.

For me, my first alert starts with my ears loudly ringing.

Sometimes I'm too busy, working too hard or having a lot of fun to hear it or I just don't want to listen. So, then my second alert kicks in (lower lip goes numb) with a fury. Now I know I'm screwing up, so I automatically start drinking a lot of water and begin the *Deep Breathing Exercise* (which lowers your blood pressure) and I find a quite place until the alerts go away. Then, I can safely go home and try to figure out what triggered the spike in my blood pressure.

Here's a few links to increase your knowledge:

http://www.chatelaine.com/health/why-you-should-stop-eating-sugar-now/

https://www.youtube.com/user/ForksOverKnives

I highly recommend!

http://www.medicaldaily.com/how-red-meat-affects-your-health-7-reasons-avoid-beef-253727

I am a
Wellness Warrior.

Here's how you do it … it is a full life style change.
A refreshing one at that!

Here is how I begin my day: I slow down! I set my alarm 30 minutes earlier than I would normally, so I'm not hurrying myself. When I first wake up I drink water, I do stretching exercises. I stretch like a cat, a dog or a bird for a few minutes and produce a big smile whether I want to or not. At first I felt like a knucklehead lying in bed with a big smile on my face, however I felt more invigorated while smiling and I am always in a little bit better mood. If you smile for just 2 minutes it will change your attitude. I do all of this instead of jumping out of bed and racing to work.

This includes pulling my knee to my chest one at a time with my hands, while pushing out with my knee as hard as I can for 5 seconds, basically a resistance type exercise. Here is a YouTube example:

https://www.youtube.com/watch?v=9hVZ4rc2_3Y
Very Important!

Link for deep breathing . . . very important as well:
https://www.youtube.com/watch?v=KNA49dhqV-w

If you speak to a superior source, let's call him or her . . . God, now is a good time for a conversation while you're still waking up. I pray for me, my family then my friends. I end it with everyone else in the world, including the bad people.

Again, the first thing that goes into your stomach everyday is water. That's right, water to wake up your stomach, like splashing water in your face:
http://www.healthyfoodhouse.com/see-happens-drink-water-empty-stomach/

Then have yourself a cup of green tea because you . . . OH . . . I almost forgot . . . you quit drinking coffee. Changing to green tea is very easy. If you find the idea challenging, start with a cup of coffee every other day. Begin alternating tea/coffee, then two days of tea and one-day coffee. Try the green tea with honey and hopefully you will enjoy it some day.

http://www.healthyfoodhouse.com/see-happens-drink-water-empty-stomach/

Don't get me wrong; I have to have that "Non fat Vanilla Latte" maybe 4-5 times a year. When I get one, it's like I'm on vacation. Nobody move . . . I'm drinking my coffee. However, green tea is better for you.

It's time for that 20-minute walk . . . we will talk about exercise later.

Next, take a long hot shower everyday. Enjoy those extra moments of solitude. Imagine your in a rain forest or under a waterfall, then put the shower jet spray on pulse into your mouth for cleaning your teeth, take that extra moment, you'll be glad you did.

I believe it's extremely important to keep up on current events. It keeps the brain in motion. I sit down for 5-10 minutes and check the Internet for the news . . . No TV. Then it's breakfast and out the door. I know some people turn on the news just for background noise. However, in my opinion, it's not good for you to listen to all those commercials regarding food to start your day. It has turned into a sport for me to dodge all those advertisements that are thrown in my face while surfing the Internet.

If you are working from home or retired, figure out a way to sweat then take the shower. Remember . . . men sweat, women glow, whatever it takes to allow your body to excrete liquid from your pores. It is yet another way of purging the toxins.

http://certification.acsm.org/blog/2013/may/the-science-of-sweat

When you drive to your first destination after leaving the house you might have a situation where you're stopped at a very long red light or someone did something outside of your "Bubble of Love" that made your blood heat up . . . so it's time for **Deep Breathing Exercise**.

Caution! There is one thing DBE can and will do to you is to put you to sleep so don't do it more than 5 times if your driving.

Now you've parked your car and, have another moment for **Deep Breathing Exercise** while walking to your destination and thanking (God) for the safe journey you just had. Yes . . . you can walk, pray and **Deep Breathing Exercise** at the same time. Don't forget to include the power of positive thinking (i.e.: what a wonderful day you're going to have) and then relax.

During the day someone might do something that ticks me/you off.

When it happens immediately think . . . humor. If nothing comes to mind, think of a friend or acquaintance that is funny and ask yourself what that person would say in a situation like this. This is a great example of codependency in a good way. If you still can't think of anything... kindly stare at them and think silence is golden.

Don't argue with idiots because they will drag you down to their level and then beat you with experience. —Greg King

While you are driving home . . . it's the same as driving to your first destination, relax. When you get home, it's hobby time. You don't watch TV anymore. Oh . . . I almost forgot . . . you might want to cancel your cable TV . . . sorry, we'll discuss TV in Chapter 12.

Don't forget to thank God for the safe journey home.

This is the ideal time to remember humor because this is when you will want/crave some food that's not good for you. So start chopping vegetables for a delicious salad. I find it very relaxing to prepare and cook in the evening because I get lost in thoughts of nothing... a might relax'n. Now that you have had that wonderful salad it's time for the hobby, play with the kids, a book, just something on the positive train of thought. I like food fast when I'm hungry, so I make up 5 or 6 salads in one large container, leaving the avocado out, then put a paper towel on top so it doesn't get soggy.

Now it's bedtime. I have a number of ways to go to sleep. My favorite is reading a book until I fall asleep or I love to play poker on my phone. Next thing you know I'm sleeping. If you're not falling asleep like you think you should . . . it's time for the **Deep Breathing Exercise** and you <u>will</u> fall asleep.

So you are saying to yourself . . . I tried that and it doesn't work. My question is "what caused you to fall off track?" Whatever it was start over and you will wake up later saying to yourself . . . "It really works".

Chapter 5 –

The Power of Self-Healing

If you believe you can heal yourself . . . you can . . . if you don't believe, you won't, so stop reading this and go buy a comfortable rock'n chair.

The power of positive thinking is the largest item in your life. You can't buy it you have to live it. Abilities wither under faultfinding, blossom under encouragement. I know I'm healing myself . . . whether I'm right or wrong.

Keeping the mind and spirit at peace is crucial to fighting cancer. Your mind has powerful influence over your physical self. Does this sound like "pseudo-science" to you? The medical community thought so for many decades. Heck, so did I for a long while. However, new research is finding a measurable connection between your thoughts and healing.

The mind-body connection is real. Researchers believe that patients who have high expectations that they will get better, their bodies will actually release biological chemicals to simulate the effect, altering specific regions of the brain to achieve the believed results. Your body has the ability to mimic the effect of antidepressants, anti-inflammatory drugs, painkillers, and even asthma medication. Much of the science behind the phenomenon may be largely unknown but that does not make it any less valid. The truth is that scientists are beginning to understand how the brain communicates with the body right down to the cellular level. An understanding of the cellular steps has blossomed since Sir John Vane won his Nobel Prize in 1982. In fact, four more Nobel Prizes have been won in the last decade on how cells communicate with each other in the body. – Source:

http://thetruthaboutcancer.com/using-mind-fight-cancer/ - sthash.pNOCho9u.dpuf

You have to accept the fact that in every major moment in your life you are alone. For example, if you are sick you can have a partner to give you some hot tea, but you are the only one who actually feels the pain. If you have to take an exam in school, your friends can support you to get ready, but in the final moment you are going to be there alone. That is going to be your success or failure. You have to deal with it.

You have to take the responsibility for the decisions you make. And at this moment you have already made a huge step toward changing your life. You are sitting in front of your computer and reading this page. You made a conscious decision to read this instead of watching TV or going out with your friends.

I cannot emphasize enough the importance of "YOU" in the process. I used "you" in this book over 600 times. It's all about you!

We are all made of energy and we are all self-healing. Eastern and ancient medical models have been based on energy for thousands of years. We witness our body's ability to heal itself when small cuts heal, and with our expectation "this will heal".

Tuning into our energy body is easy, quick and can switch our emotions and health in a few moments. When we tune into our energy bodies with our intention we can truly change our lives physically, mentally, emotionally and spiritually.

Self-healing is not at all complicated. In a few simple steps you can bring a feeling of peace into your body. You can tune into your energy body and use your thoughts and emotions to change the frequency and flow of your energy.

It is a simple as changing the channel from a negative reporting news channel to your favorite comedy show and feeling yourself relax with that change. Your day can move in a new direction that will guarantee you are inviting ease, flow and even "miracles" into your life.

So here's five easy steps you can do in five minutes. Please read through all steps and then take the next five minutes to put the wheels in motion and practice!

1) Sit in a comfortable position and become aware of your breathing. No need to change it – just pay attention to the flow – in and out, in and out. No judging it, no changing it – just noticing. This is simply becoming "present" and stopping some of the never-ending thoughts from interfering for the next few minutes.

2) Take your hands (palms together) in front of you and rub them together quickly for 30 – 60 seconds. Let them become warm from the friction and feel that warmth. Invite a slight smile in as you are rubbing your hands and taking this time. Smiling itself is healing and has the ability to switch our moods in a few seconds.

3) Hold your hands six-eight inches away from each other, facing each other and feel the energy flowing through them. This energy is always here –

you are feeling it now because of the intention and the awakening your awareness to it. As you feel this energy tune into it. Know this is part of you. Keep on smiling – doesn't this feel cool?

4) Close your eyes. See if you can move the energy up your arms, through your body. There is no "wrong way" to do this. You are awakening your energy body with your intent and your intent is to feel and to heal.

See if you can move that energy to whatever part of your body you may have some stress or disease in. Keep it there knowing you are sending it love and positive "healing energy". If you feel like you are losing touch with feeling the energy – rub your hands together again. There is no judgment and no way to do this wrong. You can picture the energy however feels right for you. Perhaps you just want to feel it; maybe you want to picture it as a white light – it is whatever way feels the easiest for you. Let yourself play with this step and smile while doing it.

5) Continue to work with this flow of energy. Call it to different parts of your body. Notice how it feels as it reaches different spaces. Know that this energy can help those areas that usually bring

you pain and feel the gratitude for finally recognizing this inherent ability in you.

Notice the energy relaxing the parts of the body it flows into. Thank your body for being able to awaken this awareness and healing. Playing with this energy flow for even five minutes can bring a state of joy and peace that you felt was impossible even minutes earlier.

How did that feel? I know when I first felt this energy I was pretty amazed that it was always present in my body yet I had not been in tune to it.

In five minutes you can change your energy flow and state of being. You can offer your body, mind and spirit some healing. Your intention along with you dedicating the five minutes to yourself is a great gift that your body, mind and soul will thank you for!

Source: http://www.finerminds.com/mind-power/self-healing-five-steps/

Releasing and transforming negative emotion while relating to feelings in a way that allows you to feel a sense of personal choice is a form of self-healing.

I use a technique for healing negative feelings on the emotional level: I think about the last time I did something that caused an accident that broke a friend's expensive vase and how bad I felt afterward. Now take that same situation and think of a way to prevent that from every happening again then I consider how I can turn it into a funny story. If your anything like me it will stick with you for a long time and there is nothing you can do about it, it's in the past. Read more: http://www.ehow.com/way_5651946_self-healing-techniques.html

Deep Breathing Exercise will oxygenate your good cells, which makes them more effective to help in the fight against the cancer cells.

Take time to smell the Air! I say "air" instead of Roses because "Sometimes there's nary a Rose Bush around."

As stated by the Peace Wellness Group, Naturopathic physicians follow three precepts to ensure their patients' safety:

Use low-risk procedures and healing compounds—such as dietary supplements, herbal extracts and homeopathy—with few or no side effects.

When possible, do not suppress symptoms, which are the body's efforts to self-heal. For example, the body may cook up a fever in reaction to a bacterial infection. Fever creates an inhospitable environment for the harmful bacteria, thereby destroying it. Of course, the naturopathic physician would not allow the fever too get dangerously high.

Customize each diagnosis and treatment plan to fit each patient. We all heal in different ways and the naturopathic physician respects our differences. Source: Peace Wellness Group.

Here are some tips to **lower your blood pressure without medication**:

1. **Go for power walks** Get a vigorous cardio workout of at least 30 minutes on most days of the week. Try increasing speed or distance so you keep challenging your ticker.

2. **Breathe deeply** Slow breathing and meditative practices. Try 5 minutes in the morning and at night. Inhale deeply and expand your belly. Exhale and release all of your tension.

3. **Potassium rich foods** Loading up on potassium-rich fruits and vegetables is an important part of

any blood pressure lowering. Top sources of potassium-rich produce include sweet potatoes, tomatoes, orange juice, potatoes, bananas, kidney beans, peas, cantaloupe, honeydew melon, and dried fruits such as prunes and raisins.

4. Be salt smart Season foods with spices, herbs, lemon, and salt-free seasoning blends.

5. Indulge in dark chocolate Dark chocolate varieties contain flavanols that make blood vessels more elastic.

6. Drink (a little) alcohol According to a review of 15 studies, the less you drink, the lower your blood pressure will drop—to a point. If you are going to drink, drink moderately.

7. Stop coffee When you're under stress, your heart starts pumping a lot more blood, boosting blood pressure, and caffeine exaggerates that effect.

8. Take up tea Many herbal teas contain hibiscus; look for blends that list it near the top of the chart of ingredients

9. Work (a bit) less Putting in more than 41 hours per week at the office raises your risk of **hypertension** by 15%.

10. Relax with music Need to bring down your

blood pressure a bit more than medication or lifestyle changes can do alone? The right tunes can help.

Meditation is a technique that is used for healing to provide space and clarity about a person's core essence and who he/she thinks he/she is.

Chapter 6 -

It's Not What You Eat

It's not about what you eat or drink . . . it's what you excrete. That solid waste is made up of dead cells, leftover indigestible fiber, bacteria and other stuff I don't know of. As you know, your food is processed in your intestines, which are lined with some very smart cells. These cells allow essential nutrients, such as sugars, amino acids, fats, vitamins and minerals to be absorbed into your bloodstream. The waste is shuttled through the rest of your digestive system, out of your body and into the toilet.

Exercise helps stimulate the natural contractions of your intestines. It also tones the muscles in your core that help create healthy elimination. Gentle activities such as taking a walk or yoga can help ease constipation, but moderate aerobic activity on a regular basis is a more effective way to keep constipation at bay in the long run.

The more veggie's I eat the faster I poop. This is another opportunity for the **Deep Breathing Exercise** stuff while your sitting on the throne.

Bowel transit time is the term doctors use to

describe how long it takes for food to pass from your mouth to your anus. Bowel transit time varies from person to person.

Vegetarians tend to have faster transit times than non-vegetarians, according to a study published in the "British Journal of Nutrition" in 1981. In this study, the distribution of transit times for non-vegetarians was between 31 hours and 96 hours. The transit times for vegetarians ranged from 27 hours to 54 hours. The average transit time for the vegetarian group was nearly 24 hours faster than for non-vegetarians.

Chapter 7 –

Risk vs. Gain

The beauty of my plan is; if you screw up for a week or a month and your cancer returns all you have to do is start over with your "new eating arrangement".

However, this time you might not get any cheat days.

I personally don't want to take that chance.

I went through a period of cheating; I reduced my veggies from 85% to 50% and everything changed. For example, when I sat down for that really nice steak dinner my shoulders and wrists were hurting while cutting it. This pain happened within a week's time. I was happy to go back to the 85%. This can and will happen to you as well. I know someday I'll drop to the 50% again then bounce back up to that wonderful 85%. It's normal to sometimes want a burger and that's ok because your body will have these cravings. Listen to what your body tells you. Get those cravings out of the way; you won't undo everything regarding your "new eating arrangement".

My first revelation was . . . I can still eat anything I want within reason, except dairy products. I will not cheat with dairy products. I still have a steak now and then but not as often as I used to.

Another trick: if you're watching a movie and a guy takes a big bite out of a juicy, dripping wet, succulent burger, now all we really want is a juicy burger. This means get in the car, buy a burger right now or we will not be able to do anything for the rest the day or night. However, I know Friday night is my night to go out and I can have anything I want . . . all I have to do is wait. I use this to get past the hankering.

You need to recognize what your body is saying to you after you eat. Fifteen minutes after I eat I listen for symptoms. Do I have a headache, a stomachache or ringing ears? If the answer is yes to any of these, you have discovered an allergic reaction to the food or ingredient. All you have to do is decipher which item it was and never consume it again.

Chapter 8 -

Exercise

I begin with push outs, meaning push your chair out and get away from the table. This equates to eating smaller portions.

Let's face it: it's not all that difficult to start a fitness routine. After all, most of us have done it more than once.

The trouble, of course, comes with sticking with it. All too often, our initial enthusiasm and energy wanes, we get distracted by other things going on in our lives, or we don't think we're seeing results quickly enough -- and we throw in the towel.

Yet many people do manage to hang in there, and would no sooner skip their regular workout than their morning shower. What's their secret?

A recent study by researcher Diane Klein, PhD, shed some light on the subject. Long-term exercisers (who had been working out for an average of 13 years) were asked to rank what motivated them to keep up with their regimes.

Their answers might surprise you. The exercisers were not as concerned with powerful pecks and awesome abs as they were with feeling good and being healthy.

Here's how the study participants ranked their motivators:

- Fitness
- Feelings of well-being
- Enjoyment of the exercise
- Making exercise a priority
- Sleeping better
- Feeling alert
- Being relaxed
- Appearance

So, once you have your priorities in the right place, how can you become one of the fitness faithful?

I have compiled a few tips for making fitness a habit in your life.

1. Do a variety of activities you enjoy. And remember, there's no rule that says you have to go to a gym or buy equipment. I like sit-ups (in bed), walking and riding my bicycle is my form of exercise/activities. It's also great for my lower back when it is sore.

2. Commit to another person. The social aspect of

exercise is important for me, I use to drive by a friend's house on the way to the racquetball court, and pick him up at 5:30 am. If he wasn't ready, that constituted a $100 fine which I never had to collect. I won't let the other person down.

3. Make exercise a priority. "It has to be a non-negotiable,"

Encourage yourself every day to do a little tiny bit better today than yesterday.

Chapter 9 –

PH Balance

My wellness Doctor told me I had to raise my PH level and start drinking water that has a +9 PH value. I bought the only water I could find with a 9+ PH on the label, which was very expensive and drank it for a few months.

With the inquiring mind I am blessed with, I bought a Digital PH Meter Tester Pocket Portable ($10 on ebay) and tested everything from the 9+ bottled water, through all the different bottled waters from four different grocery stores and the tap water from my home. The results really surprised me, the 9+ results came in the lowest at 6.8, so I stopped buying that expensive crap, The grocery stores averaged at 8.5 and my tap water came in at the highest . . . 9.0. I have read articles regarding tap water having fluoride and chlorine so I suggest if you are concerned of contaminants risk in your tap water, obtain a copy of your city's annual water quality report (they are mandated by law) and review it with your physician.

Personally I have found the grocery store sells a case of bottled water for around $3 and I will continue to buy and test the bottled water at least once a month, which I believe to be very important.

Dr. Otto H. Warburg is a Nobel Prize winner and has spent his entire life in an effort to find the cause of cancer. He strongly believed that there was a direct connection between the pH value and the oxygen level. Any pH value higher than 7.365 is alkaline and is followed by a higher concentration of oxygen molecules, and lower pH value, which is acidic, means lower oxygen level . . . and healthy cells need that oxygen to survive. You can buy PH strips on the Internet to check on your personal PH   level.

In 1931 Dr. Warburg received the Nobel Prize in Medicine for his amazing discovery. He outlined, "Cancerous tissues are acidic, whereas healthy tissues are alkaline. Water splits into H+ and OH- ions, if there is an excess of H+, it is acidic; if there is an excess of OH- ions, then it is alkaline". 'Deprive a cell 35% of its oxygen for 48 hours and it may become cancerous." And don't forget **Deep Breathing Exercises.**

Dr. Warburg's study showed that oxygen deficiency is the root cause of cancer, meaning that acidity increases as the levels of oxygen decrease. He also found that cancer cells are anaerobic (do not breathe oxygen) and cannot thrive in aerobic conditions, or in an alkaline state.

See more at:
http://www.healthyfoodhouse.com/the-root-cause-of-cancer-and-why-has-it-been-kept-a-secret/#sthash.fLNo8csF.dpuf

Foods that raise your body pH (i.e., are alkaline-producing), from highest to lowest are vegetable juice, parsley, raw spinach, broccoli, celery, garlic, barley, dried figs, raisins, herb teas, lemon water, stevia, carrots, green and lima beans, beets, lettuce, carob, dates, grapes, papaya, kiwi, berries, apples, pears, hazelnuts, almonds, green tea, maple syrup, squash, asparagus, tomato, mushrooms, onions, cabbage, peas, cauliflower, olives, coconut, oranges, cherries, pineapple, peaches, avocados, lentils, quinoa, goat milk and cheese, chestnuts, brazil nuts, flax seeds, olive oil, ginger and raw honey. All of the above items constitute your shopping list at the grocery.

Read more about you PH. Source :
http://www.ehow.com/about_5487572_foods-raise-body-ph.html

"Join the Body Balance Revolution Now!"
http://www.phbodybalance.com

We are alkaline by design, but acid by function (breathing, digesting, thinking . . .the list goes on) and many of our beverages and foods today are very acidic, finger pointing fast foods, sodas, coffee, and the list goes on. So as a result of poor diets, degraded food, water, and air, consequently we've become too acidic.

How do we help ourselves? First I suggest targeting your acidic hot spots. What's causing you the most incoming acid? Then, create an exchange or a shortcut to diffuse that acid, one you will be happy with and that can become a part of your everyday habit. At the same time we can work on some fundamental foundational changes that will enhance your alkalinity.

Perspective: If you can shift your perspective of food and water from simply being fuel and hydration, and develop your understanding of "you are what you eat" meaning "maintenance and healing comes from what we ingest", you will begin to understand why we, as a world, have become too acidic.

Fortunately we can control our own environments. The key is to know what is most important, how to convert acid into acid busters, and simply make "Small Changes That Make The Biggest

Differences" - that you like better, taste better, and are better for you. Our pH measurement is a health marker we have control over. Testing your body fluid with pH test strips is a simple way to measure your internal fluids.

pH Scale: (acid) 0 - 14 (alkaline)   Optimal: Saliva 7.365 / Urine 6.8

pH balance or optimal health can be achieved when our blood and tissues are pH neutral, i.e., our bodies are nourished and hydrated and we rid our bodies of waste and toxins.

Cause and effect - Most of us are struggling with performance or feeling "sick and tired", are over or under weight, maybe obese, experiencing health challenges of many degrees, or we know people that are. It's all around us, and the most common denominators are degraded food, water and air.

If you believe you are what you eat, what you drink, and what you breathe, then know we are for the most part, a result of our environment. Fortunately we can control our own personal environments, adjust to the conditions, and make "Small Changes That Make Big Differences".

Source: http://www.phbodybalance.com

Chapter 10 –

Wording on the Labels

Everyone should know how to read labels You **may be aware** of some of the following tricks, lies, schemes and plots to keep people malnourished and in need of constant medical attention, but then again, you may not. The biggest lies in this world are the ones more likely to be believed, and "Big Food" has that kind of money to spend on you, so here we go:

"For added freshness" and **"as a preservative"** -- These *preservatives* kill fungus and mutate human cells into cancer, yet these slogans are seen on bread all over the world and on jar labels for just about everything.

"As a preservative . . ." -- Sodium benzoate* is a chemical used to stave off fungus from growing in foods, and for the molds that kill taste and spoil goods on the shelf sooner. Unfortunately for humans, it deprives cells of oxygen. Fungus killers and mold inhibitors can also deteriorate the myelin sheath -- the cellular structure that insulates nerve cells. Don't be fooled by tricky Big Food slogans. (*While benzoic acid is found naturally in low levels in many fruits, the sodium benzoate listed on a product's label is synthesized in a lab!)

"**All natural**" -- Means absolutely nothing. If you think that these words change anything about the quality of the product, you are gravely mistaken. The FDA has no parameters of health here.

Pasteurized -- Means cooked quickly at high heat and "cooks" the nutrition right out. That's why "Big Milk" (dairy industry) tries to shut down farmers of organic, raw milk, because people might catch on that nutrients, when actually in food, can do a body good. Batch or "vat" is the simplest and oldest method of pasteurization, which heats the milk to over 150 degrees Fahrenheit! This kills enzymes, probiotics and nutrients. Raw food experts will tell you that most food cooked at 118 degrees becomes useless. And adding back some (dead) vitamin D to milk is also another ploy to confuse the people who find out what pasteurization really means. Most orange juice is pasteurized. Hint, hint!

Fortified -- Cooked, dead vitamins are added "back in" to a product (useless) so the manufacturer can make false health claims to make junk food sound better. Hence the popular lingo for kids' cereals.

RDA -- "Recommended Daily Allowance" -- Of what? Of dead food, GMO food, hormone-laden food, conventional milk, meat, cheese and wheat gluten? Dirty dozen fruits and vegetables? That's cancer food -- so tell us again, *what's the daily recommended allowance of cancer food*?

Farm-raised -- This means the fish "farmers" breed fish in a pond or indoor tank system where they can create unnatural breeds that are larger and give them hormones to make bigger (cancerous) fish for profits.

GMO is not even labeled in the US (except for a few choice states, soon). Talk about tricky! How about tricking people into eating genetically MUTATED food that's corrupt with pesticide, insecticide and herbicide?
Source: http://www.naturalnews.com

Super Tricky Lingo

There is "no significant difference" between milk from cows given rbST, or rbGH, and regular milk . . . this industry lingo is to cover up the fact that **artificial** and **synthesized Growth Hormones** given to cows to make them fatter or produce TOO MUCH MILK also cause health detriment for humans that consume that milk, cheese, yogurt, etc. This hormone, rbST (recombinant somatotropin) -- also called rbGH (recombinant bovine growth hormone) -- increases the amount of IGF-1 in milk, a chemical that has been linked to certain **cancers**.

Source:
http://www.naturalnews.com/046894_food_industry_marketing_claims_GMOs.html?utm_content=buffer2740e&utm_medium=social&utm_source=facebook.com&utm_campaign=buffer

Chapter 11 –

Is Cow's Milk Pure?

"MILK" Just the word itself sounds comforting! "How about a nice cup of hot milk?" The last time you heard that question it was from someone who cared for you--and you appreciated their effort. The entire matter of food and especially that of milk is surrounded with emotional and cultural importance. Milk was our very first food. If we were fortunate it was our mother's milk. Please read the full article courtesy of Dr. Kradjian http://www.notmilk.com/kradjian.html

Lets talk about IGF-1, This is some bad stuff you need to know about so I'll start with the definition:

IGF-1
Insulin-like growth factor I, somatomedin-C A polypeptide hormone structurally similar to proinsulin, synthesized in the liver and fibroblasts, giving fibroblasts a paracrine function; serum levels correlate with development of 2° sex characteristics in puberty ↑ in Acromegaly, gigantism ↓ in starvation, anorexia nervosa, African pygmies, ↓ somatomedins, Laron dwarfism, kwashiorkor. Liver dieses in children, GH

deficiency, hypopituitarism.

Did you understand all of this? Me neither, all I know is it's very bad for you and our government doesn't care or they would change it.

Now I would like to share the timeline starting 45 years ago without our knowledge:

1979 Scientists discovered IGF-I.

1989 Scientists learned that IGF-I was an identical match in the cow's body and the human body.

1994 FDA encountered the biggest controversy in their history by approving the genetically engineered bovine growth hormone known as BGH (aka BST). When that hormone is injected into cows, levels of IGF-I in milk increase by about 80%.

1998 IGF-I was called the key factor in the growth and proliferation of prostate cancer (Science - January, 1998) and breast cancer (The Lancet - May, 1998).
WOW . . . **Sixteen years ago!**

1999 IGF-I was identified as the key factor in the

growth of lung cancer (Journal of the National Cancer Institute - January, 1999).
WOW . . . **Fifteen years ago!**

The Journal of the American Dietetic Association (Page 1231) said this about IGF-I levels in people who drink milk:

"Serum IGF-I levels (blood levels) increased significantly in the milk group . . . an increase of about 10% above baseline--but was unchanged in the control group." Source:
http://www.notmilk.com/igf1time.txt

STOP MILK . . . This link has great substitutes for milk:
http://thescienceofeating.com/proteins/stop-drinking-milk/

I hear from a lot of people regarding the calcium in milk is so important for their children, I say "there's calcium in broccoli and those cows with the big strong bones don't drink milk". Cows eat a plant-based food.This link below gives you a list of Nondairy Foods with Calcium:

http://pediatrics.about.com/od/calcium/a/06_calcium_food.htm?utm_term=list high calcium foods&utm_content=p1-main-1-

Calcium? Where do the COWS get calcium for their big strong bones . . . from plants! Hmmmm!

Society stresses the importance of calcium, but rarely magnesium. Yet, magnesium is vital to enzymatic activity. In addition to insuring proper absorption of calcium, magnesium is critical to proper neural and muscular function and to maintaining proper pH balance in the body. Magnesium, along with vitamin B6 (pyridoxine), helps to dissolve calcium phosphate stones, which often accumulate from excesses of dairy intake. Good sources of magnesium include beans, green leafy vegetables like kale and collards, whole grains and orange juice. Non-dairy sources of calcium include green leafy vegetables, almonds, asparagus, broccoli, cabbage, oats, beans, parsley, sesame seeds and tofu. Source: notmilk.com

Chapter 12 –

Cancel Your Television

I am angry with the cable companies and TV manufacturers for making me not wanting to exercise or play outside. Lack of exercise kills millions more than polio.
Learn more, this is a great article:
http://www.naturalnews.com/048588_Arizona_cardiologist_measle_vaccine_immunization_chemicals.html#ixzz3RTWSOBqC

I highly recommend you cancel your TV/Cable contract. You say . . . whaaaaaa, seriously? What I'm going to explain to you is how to change your life for the better. Watch this link below to see a common mass media trick:

https://video.search.yahoo.com/video/play;_ylt=A2KIo.DIRW5Uu1kAnbP7w8QF;_ylu=X3oDMTByZWc0dGJtHNlYwNzcgRzbGsDdmlkBHZ0aWQDBGdwb3MDMQ?p=the+secrets+of+food+marketing&vid=2f2f26c9fe6427c7cb524225e3818a58&l=7%3A00&turl=http%3A%2F%2Fts2.mm.bing.net%2Fth%3Fid%3DVN.608020661990852189%26pid%3D15.1&rurl=http%3A%2F%2Fwww.youtube.com%2Fwatch%3Fv%3DmKTORFmMycQ&tit=eTalks+-

This is all about how you were/are brainwashed regarding the food you eat. When I go to someone's house that has the TV on, all I hear are the commercials that foster eating foods that are not good for you.

"It's time for your Burger and Cannnnnndy Bar . . . but don't forget the energy drinnnnnnnnk".

As you know, there are companies out there that have streaming videos or CDs you can rent. I stopped watching TV 6 years ago not because of cancer, but because one night (while paying $120 a month) I surfed channels for 2 hours trying to relax, then it hit me there's nothing worth watching. I then heard this voice in my head say "Geeeeeetttt Riiiiiid ooooof Yourrrrrrr TVs." The next day I gave my TV's away and it was the best thing I did for myself that year.

For example, turn on the news tomorrow morning with a stopwatch in hand for one hour. Start the stop watch when you hear a news story, not some story coming up or in our next half hour but a news story then stop it . . . you will be amazed on what

74

enters your brain that is allegedly not good for you. Count how many food references are on the morning news.

My Father told me "you need to stay up on current events". I still do that on the Internet and I get to pick and choose from the headlines.

So as soon as your TV contract is up, CANCEL it. You will not be sorry.

Chapter 13 –

Summation

When it comes to everyday life and the new eating arrangement, you'll find it rewarding to look at your journal and see what you have accomplished. Yay!

Realize you're breaking one life style and beginning a new healthier one. This is a major commitment and a rewarding one as well. Fact: it takes 21 days to break a habit; this is if you stop cold turkey. If you cheat, you start the 21 days all over again and don't worry; you have the rest of your life to get it right.

If you have to have a sandwich buy the Sandwich Thins bread. Add a nice avocado, onion, lettuce and garlic, so you can have a taste of bread. You conquer the urge and have a sandwich, then give the rest of the bread away.

I have suggested eating anything you want twice a week. Let's break it down: 3 meals a day, 7 days a week equates to 21 meals a week. Two of them are special . . .

Let's say you were to start off eliminating 1 of the 5 items mentioned in Chapter 4 for 21 days.

1. Dairy products, anything from a cow
2. Meat by-products
3. Fried foods
4. Wheat
5. Sugar

Dairy Products, as I mentioned before, is the number one cancer causing product on the market, in my opinion. It is the best starting point then go in the order that I have listed above. Breaking the 21-day habit for each of the 5 items one at a time is 105 days. This equates to a little over three months to accomplish. I stopped all 5 items at once because I thought this is the proper way to do it and I was miserable. In hindsight, I recommend you spread the love over 105 days.

Let's say you stopped all items overnight and after 12 days you couldn't sit still because you wanted a burger or ice cream . . . outside of the "every 10th meal". You got in your car, drove down at 11:30 at night, got the burger enjoyed the heck out it and as your driving home you start to feel guilty . . . STOP! Look at your journal and realize you went 12 days . . . Yay!

Go home satisfied and then write the burger in the journal. When you wake up the next morning knowing your going back on schedule today think about what happened and why. When it starts happening again in two nights you can curb it by brushing your teeth, working on a hobby or watching a movie, etc. Remember, you have made a difference and your working hard on the **"it's a new eating arrangement!"**

Once you start feeling more energy and less pain you will want more. Your commitment will grow stronger with the "anything you want every 10th meal".

Continue reading books regarding this subject (i.e. The China Study & Forks Over Knifes). It is very motivational to say the least and helps you stay on track. Hence, "Get Off The Cow Now!"

Let Us Review!

- Get Off the Cow Now!
- Get on the THC, Medical Marijuana.
- Find a Wellness Doctor and become a Flexitarian
- Start cutting down sugar until it's over.
- Set two times a week where you can eat anything and stick to it.
- Don't worry if you screw up . . . you can start over today.
- Quit feeding Jok.
- Keep an eye out for new ideas for your salads.
- **Deep Breathing Exercise** . . . every time you think of it, very important!
- If you have meat, have 20% meat and 80% Veggies!
- Watch the Film Forks Over Knifes . . . very important.
- The 4 F's for Good Poops.
- The 5 F's for Good Living: Fair, Firm, Frank, Friendly & Forgiving.
- It's important to pray for yourself!
- Relax
- Adopt a whole foods plant base diet.
- YOUR FOOD IS YOUR MEDICINE
- PH Balance is very important.

Keep educating yourself on your bodily intake.

Eight principles of food and health

The authors of the book "China Study" describe their eight principles of food and health:

- Nutrition represents the combined activities of countless food substances. The whole is greater than the sum of its parts.
- Vitamin supplements are not a panacea for good health.
- There are virtually no nutrients in animal-based foods that are not better provided by plants.
- Genes do not determine disease on their own. Genes function only by being activated, or expressed, and nutrition plays a critical role in determining which genes, good and bad, are expressed.
- Nutrition can substantially control the adverse effects of noxious chemicals.
- The same nutrition that prevents disease in its early stages can also halt or reverse it in its later stages.
- Nutrition that is truly beneficial for one chronic disease will support health across the board.
- Good nutrition creates health in all areas of our existence. All parts are interconnected.[13] Source: The China study

Below I have put together a four-week menu just for you!

First Week Menu at 60% Flexitarian

Breakfast   Lunch   Dinner

Mon.__Cereal_____Salad_____**Stir Fry Vegies**

Tues.__Shake___Sandwich_Fish

Wed.__Anything__Salad____**Stir Fry Vegies**

Thurs._Cereal_____Salad___Salad

Fri._____Shake_____Salad___Steak

Sat.___Shake_____Salad__Salad

Sun.___Omelette___Burger_Salad

If you feel better after one week, stick with this menu above. If you want to feel better than that, try to eliminate the fish on Tuesday and the burger on Sunday. You have two weeks to reach the goal of 80%.

Fourth Week Menu at 80% Flexitarian

Breakfast Lunch   Dinner

Mon.__Cereal___Salad____Stir Fry Vegies

Tue.__Shake_____Salad_____Salad

Wed.__Anything__Salad____Stir Fry Vegies

Thurs._Cereal____Salad___Salad

Friday__Shake_____Salad__Steak & Lobster

Sat____Shake_____Salad___Salad

Sunday__Omelette__Sandwich_Salad

If you find you need more meat, feel free to eat it for it will shorten your life by a few hours or a day, so . . . what the heck, you only live once and of course, it's just my opinion!

This is not a diet . . .
"it's a new eating arrangement!"

Discover the variety of all vegetarian, vegan foods and cooking ideas. For recipes and cookbooks, go to www.upc-online.org/recipes/.

Thank you for your time.

Most importantly . . .
"All the Best!"

List of Wonderful Contributors in alphabetical order:
Wendy Alcala
Elizabeth Foley
Gail Stepanek

treatment and advice of a qualified licensed medical professional. This site offers people medical information and tells them their alternative medical options, but in no way should anyone consider that this book represents the "practice of medicine." This book assumes no responsibility for how this material is used. Also note that this ebook frequently updates its contents, due to a variety of reasons, therefore, some information may be out of date. The statements regarding alternative treatments for cancer have not been evaluated by the FDA.

ISBN-13:
978-1508663676

ISBN-10:
150866367X